The Ultimate Fat Loss Guide:

Fat Loss Secrets

Boost Metabolism And Finally Get Lean And Ripped, Lose Fat And Get Shredded Fast With These Simple Fat Loss Secrets!

I0428332

Chris Smith

STOP!!! Before you read any further....Would you like to know the Secrets of Body Transformation?

If your answer is yes, then you are not alone. Thousands of people are looking for the secret to rapidly burn body fat, keep the weight off, become healthier, and truly transform their body and life for good.

If you have been searching for these answers without much luck, you are in the right place!

Not only will you gain incredible insight in this book, but because I want to make sure to give you as much value as possible, right now for a limited time you can get full **100% FREE access to a VIP bonus EBook** entitled **THE 7 KEYS TO BODY TRANSFORMATION!**

Just Go Here For Free Instant Access:

www.liveFitVIP.com

Legal Notice

Disclaimer Notice

Table Of Contents

Introduction

I want to thank you and congratulate you for purchasing the book, *"Fat Loss Secrets: The Ultimate Fat Loss Guide! - Boost Metabolism And Finally Get Lean And Ripped, Lose Fat And Get Shredded Fast With These Simple Fat Loss Secrets!"*.

This book contains proven steps and strategies on how to lose fat and get the body you have always dreamed of!

Over the years, countless fad diets have come and gone. Along with the fad diets came the supplements. At first, some of the supplements seemed like they could be of benefit to you and healthy for you to consume, but as time has gone on so has the supplement industry. Supplements are now chemically engineered magic potion pills. Some of them do help you lose body fat, but at what expense to your health?

It doesn't have to be this complicated! If you are tired of riding the diet roller coaster and jumping on and off the hope train of the supplement industry, then you have come to the right place. This is where, armored with the truth, you can take control of your body and achieve your dreams for good. So read this book, apply the principles, and lose the fat.

Thanks again for purchasing this book, I hope you enjoy it!

Chapter 1: The Truth About Weight Loss

If you have ever thought about losing weight then you have probably researched long and wide in search for the newest craze to shed unwanted body fat. If you have been taught by your weight loss experience that skipping solid food and jogging a lot is the only way to get the results that you want, you may be getting the entire weight loss idea wrong.

The truth about weight loss is that it is not what it seems, and people are getting the wrong kind of training when it comes to what they should do to shed extra pounds. Here is the list of some of the things that you thought are the sole reasons why people lose weight.

"Clean" and "detox" food.

Excessive movement and exercise

Staying away from junk food

Lower sugar intake

Lower amount of carbs in the diet

Eating healthy food

Refusing to eat dinner

Doing cardio exercises

Bodybuilding and gaining muscles

Using a much smaller plate

And many more fad diets and programs

These are just a few examples of an extensive list, but here's the truth about these things. While they may assist in losing weight, they are working on an entirely different concept, and so do you. In fact, you can skip all these and still lose weight, which is something that gym trainers and companies that sell healthy packed juices, pills, and potions do not tell.

Losing weight does not need to be complicated or some sort of rocket science, and even if you do not have the money to enroll in a diet/nutrition program or gym training, the ideal weight is achievable. All you need to do is pay attention to the calories that you take in, it's really that simple! Crazy! Right? After all this time we have been told that all food is not created equal, keep your carbs and fats down and you will lose weight. I won't sit here and tell you that eating vegetables and lean meats is not healthier for you than eating sugar, carbs, and fats, but from a standpoint of losing weight, the most important thing you can do is take in less calories than you burn. That's it. If they exceed the requirement your body needs to function, shed them. In this sense, losing weight is actually very straightforward.

Chapter 2: The Law Of Thermodynamics

A calorie is a calorie, no matter where you get it from. Moreover, as per the law of thermodynamics, energy is neither created, nor destroyed. It can only be transformed. That law holds true inside the body. When you have excessive calorie intake and you do not use it up, it becomes something else.

I like to compare weight loss to a bank account. If you make deposits in the account, the balance will grow, and grow, and grow. If you take withdrawals from the account then the account will get smaller, and smaller. It is very similar with weight loss. It is a constant balance between deposits and withdrawals. If you make more deposits than withdrawals, then you will gain weight. If you make less deposits than withdrawals, then you will lose weight. Any stored amount energy is stored in your body as fat, which actually functions as reserve deposits of energy.

You will continually gain weight when you consume calories that you do not burn, and they pile up in the form of fat, on top of what you already have.

Therefore, you cannot really lose fat until you lose the excess calories that you already have in your body. You should also take into consideration that no matter how fancy or healthy the food you eat, when you think about weight loss, they still yield a certain amount of calories, and the rule will still stand.

With that in mind, the only rule when it comes to losing weight is this: in order to remove the stored calories in your body, you must achieve caloric deficit.

Chapter 3: Defining Caloric Deficit

Caloric deficit simply refers to burning off more calories than what you consume, or consuming fewer calories than what you can burn. In doing so, no matter what you eat, or do, you will successfully lose weight. It is arguably not the "secret" or "trick" to weight loss – it is the only thing that works.

There is one thing that you should understand about energy. Every person has a unique amount of calories needed in order to perform daily activities and for the body to do all the physiological activities that would promote survival. If you are the type of person whose job is to sit behind a desk for 8 hours, the amount of calories you need to function well every day would differ from the requirements of a construction worker, which would most likely need more.

Scenarios of Calorie Intake

Here are the things that happen when people take in calories and use them.

If a person consumes the same amount of calories as he uses up daily, he achieves a maintenance level. That means that weight is maintained because what he gained in calories is the same as what he lost.

If a person consumes more than the amount of calories than he used, caloric surplus is achieved. That means that the unused calories would be stored in the body in the form of fat. You can call that weight gain.

If a person consumes less calories than what is actually needed to be burned for his activities, he achieves calorie deficit. Essentially, it would force the body to look for an alternative energy source, tapping the fat stored in the body. That causes weight loss.

When you think about it, if you are maintaining your current weight by eating about 3000 calories worth of food, you lose weight if you reduce it to 2500. That holds true no matter what kind of food you eat, whether it is considered healthy or not. Weight loss only happens when you start minding the calories you take in daily and compare them to your personal requirements of energy.

Chapter 4: There is Something Wrong With The Fat Loss Advertisements!

If weight loss is as simple as caloric deficit, why are companies advertising a lot of other things that promote weight loss? Why are people losing a lot of money buying expensive juices, pills, and potions made from green leafy vegetables, and trying to enroll in expensive gym classes just to trim the fat away?

Some of these supplements actually do work in regards to helping you lose weight by manipulating your body to burn more calories, ramping your heart rate up, or changing your hormone levels, etc. But the question I would ask myself if I were you is, how healthy can this be to artificially change these things in hopes of accomplishing a goal that I can without a doubt do with a simple calorie deficit? The advertisements promote that you eat only a certain kind of food every day and do a certain amount of activity and take a certain supplement, but in the end, you are led into boxing your lifestyle in such a way that you obey fads to achieve the shape that you want.

What Does Not Fit?

Of course, you may think that if losing weight is as simple as slashing off the calories, then maybe doctors would not have to research and concoct those so called healthy juices and supplements for you to buy. Maybe there is some mistake about the calories, or otherwise, they would not have to offer these magical potions in the marketplace.

But for a moment just think about fat loss as an industry instead of a simple problem with a simple solution. The fat loss industry is one of the largest in the world and ever expanding with our ever expanding waistlines and lifestyles. Do you think it would be such a vast industry if people were simply advised to eat less calories to burn off the fat - they so desire to rid themselves of? The answer is of course, no! In truth diet is a commodity that sells, but in order for it to sell the supplement companies must continue to find new solutions to the same old problem. One solution that actually solved the issue would be extremely unprofitable. Do yourself a favor, and don't ride this roller coaster of hope. Get with the truth and apply the knowledge to once and for all reach your goals.

Research Says

It seems that a simple calorie deficit being the most effective solution to fat loss is too good to believe, but there are extreme examples about weight loss that might convince you otherwise.

The Twinkie Experiment

Mark Haub, a human nutrition professor in Kansas University, wanted to prove the same thing, which is the application of the Law of Thermodynamics in the human body. To prove this, Dr. Haub embarked on a 10-week diet that is composed mainly of snack foods like Twinkies and other sugary snack meals. While these things lack nutritional value, and highly believed to be the cause of obesity, he was able to achieve caloric deficit.

He achieved it mainly by effectively reducing his calorie intake from 2600 (the estimated calorie intake for his maintenance level) to 1800, by mainly eating junk food. The experiment is something that you should not try – it is just to prove that as long as you are reducing the calorie intake and achieve a deficit, instead of a surplus, you will lose weight no matter what type of food you are eating.

What Does It Prove?

While the Twinkie Experiment is not a laudable way to lose weight, it also says that the reverse is true – eating too much healthy food will result in weight gain. The best plan of action is to eat healthy food and just mind the calorie intake in such a way that you are eating to get the right nutrition and achieve a calorie deficit. Keep in mind that no matter how healthy or clean you are eating, eating beyond what is needed by your body would still result in gaining fat. Also, keep in mind that a pound of fat in your body amounts to 3,500 calories sitting inside you.

What does it say about the fad diets that people believe in so much that they are willing to bet their money on it? As long as your goal is losing weight, what you eat does not matter. You can still achieve the same thing by eating the dirtiest food doctors advise against, but it is not smart or healthy long term. Everyone should make sure to get the proper amount of carbs, proteins, fats, and especially vegetables and fruit in their diet to make sure they are reaching all of their body's requirements and to remain healthy and active for the long term. What good would it do you to eat garbage all day to achieve and maintain a level of body fat for years, then to incur another larger problem in the form of a vital health problem. In short don't just eat badly because you can, make sure you have a balanced diet.

You don't need to invest in the latest fad or exercise program to accomplish your goal of fat loss. Instead of betting your health, happiness, and resources on things that are popular, invest in activities that will not cost you an extra dime to do. Invest in a diet and exercise plan that works according to what you need.

Chapter 5: Why Do Those Diets And Supplements Work Then?

To keep things simple, here is the only way all diets and supplements work: they indirectly cause a caloric deficit. There is no other way around that. However, let's take a look at some popular diets that can work for you, as long as you stay true to our number 1 rule - eat less calories than you burn!

South Beach Diet and Atkins Diet

South Beach and Atkins work similarly by restricting carbohydrates that you can eat, which means you should rid your diet of potatoes, rice, bread and similar carbs for the first two weeks. After that, most of these carbohydrate-laden foods are still discouraged. Unhealthy fats are also discouraged in these diets. In effect, you lose a great deal of calories you would normally get from fatty and starchy food, but you replace it with the great ones through strategic snacking. In effect, it aims for caloric deficit, and with a calorie deficit you will lose weight.

Juicing

Juicing is a pretty straightforward way to lose weight, essentially because it takes away the solids from your daily meal. Solid foods are easy way to get a lot of calories into your system. What juicing promises is a lot of fiber, and daily nutrition allowance. However, you may want to think about ordering pre-made juices, as it is regularly advertised. It is very expensive, and you can do the juice at home instead. This is definitely not a long term solution.

Food Supplements

A lot of existing popular diets come with food supplements, and the goal is for you to not lose the nutrition you need while shedding the weight. Just like diets, they work by not letting you eat too much. Still, the aim is to achieve caloric deficit.

Baby Food Diet

If there is a diet that would make you lose your appetite, it probably is the baby food diet. Arguably, it works by making you eat 14 jars of baby food, or eat three healthy adult meals and replace all snacks with baby food. A jar of baby food would yield a hundred calories a pop, and if this is the only thing you have in your refrigerator, there is no way to go but the way of shedding pounds. However, it also lacks all the nutrition that you need as an adult, and well, they do not really go well with coffee or tea. When you get the chance to eat a regular meal, you risk wanting to overeat because of hunger. In other words, it can be very difficult to tolerate it.

Calorie is King

If you carefully look at popular diets, you are essentially paying for ways to achieve a caloric deficit, but get the right nutritional value to not let your health decline. This is not a bad thing if you examine it. However, as all doctors say, there is not a single diet that will work for everybody, which means that even if you went on a diet that is trending in popularity, it does not mean that it will work or be healthy for you. Since you need a unique amount of calories and different amount of vitamins and minerals to keep your body healthy, it would be better to find a program that works for you.

It is not bad to believe in a doctor-formulated diet. In fact, there is good reason for you to, especially if the one who formulated and prescribed it is your own nutritionist and physician, who knows all about your needs. If the advice comes from somebody else's doctor, or from your television, it might not necessarily work for you. The last thing that you want to do is waste your money on useless products, but still not lose a pound.

You can create a diet and exercise regimen that will work out for your daily activities, and the type of meals that you actually want to eat. It is way simpler too, and it is guaranteed to make you feel the effects. It is called caloric deficit, and nothing else will work like it.

Chapter 6: Creating Your Personal Caloric Deficit

There are hundreds more ways for you to achieve weight loss through caloric deficit. However, there is no such thing as the perfect diet plan, unless it is your own.

Arguably, the best diet for you is the diet that is specially formulated to fit your body and lifestyle. To create a diet plan that works for you, there are two things that you have to identify first.

Your Goals

When you create a diet plan, you have a variety of goals in mind. Apart from losing fat, these would probably be included in the list:

Improve health

Gain muscles

Improve your performance at a certain sport or activity

Feel less tired, or experience less difficulty in carrying out daily tasks

Lose fat and look good, or fit into a smaller sized clothes

Identifying your specific set of goals will tell you a lot about what, how much and how frequent you should eat, it tells you about the right type of exercise you should do. It will also tell you about the things that you should quit doing, or what you should include in your existing activities.

How Many Calories?

Taking your goals into consideration, how many calories should you lose to get the results that you want? Moreover, how many calories are you used to having?

Keep in mind that if your goal is to achieve muscle gain, those things are not built out of nothing. You will need to eat a certain amount of calories to convert them into muscles. As per research, a pound of muscle is equal to about 600 calories. Also, remember that a person with body fat is more likely to get muscles and reduce fat, and that goes the opposite for a person who has less body fat. In order to avoid losing your hard earned muscles you have to do the right type of workout.

What You Are Trying To Do

To state the obvious, you can lose fat easily by eating a very little amount of food. However, doing that would leave you too hungry or too weak to carry out tasks that you can normally do. At the same time, you should keep in mind that the body can burn up fat, get rid of water, but it can also use up your muscles as energy source when it is needed. Keep in mind that losing weight is not necessarily losing fat – these are different. You are trying to lose fat, but you want to keep the things that already look good on you.

What you want to do instead is to find a certain "sweet spot" in the calorie deficit that will allow you to easily lose excess weight without making your body suffer. For athletes, that caloric deficit sweet spot is 300 to 500 calories per day. This will be different for you if you have been training your body otherwise. The sweet spot would still depend on the amount of calories you take in, the kind of food that you process for energy and body building, and the type of activities you do to burn off energy.

The Right Amount of Everything

When it comes to your goals, you are trying to get the right combination of food and workout, without avoiding the excess of anything. If you are trying to lose weight primarily, you are trying to get a diet that will make you burn stored fat, without making you feel hungry too soon.

Yes, there are certain kinds of food that would give you the benefit of burning the fat, while keeping your muscles intact. Protein is known to be the building block of muscle. Eating food that is rich in protein is known to be the most convenient way to eat while losing fat – it does not matter when you eat it, as long as you are getting an adequate amount of this nutrient. At the same time, it makes you feel less hungry over a long time. Ideally, you eat one gram of protein per pound of body weight.

Excessive exercise is also something that you should avoid. If you are burning way too many calories than your body will choose to use up your muscles instead.

If you are beginning to lose weight, go on maintenance workouts and lift your choice of weight to promote strength. If you are doing bench presses for 150 lbs., continue to try to use this amount of weight for bench presses during the entire fat loss process. Maintaining the strength that you have is necessary to maintain your muscles.

However, keep in mind that achieving caloric deficit is actually decreasing the energy you have in your body. While you are embarking on this entire fat loss process, you are also decreasing your body's ability to recover, even to perform. If you feel that you are too tired for a workout, or you feel that you are experiencing pain, do not overdo it. Lessen the frequency or the intensity of exercise and let your body catch up with your goals first.

You may also think that the best way to lose fat is to cut the calories in big amounts. Do not even think about it. Cutting down a big chunk of calories that you are used to having would make your personal fat loss regimen hard to maintain, and it would make you feel that trimming the fat off is a painful process. Keep the calorie loss in moderation, so that you can enjoy the benefits without having to suffer too much for it.

Chapter 7: Getting The Best Results

Now that getting rid of excess fat is simpler and more cost-effective, it seems that you will be able to reach your goals, which is to get lean with muscles, and ultimately say goodbye to ugly fat deposits. However, you can still do better than that.

Keep in mind that while you are going through all the workouts and cutting your calorie intake, you are also trying to achieve a healthy body. It would still be best to consult with your personal dietician or physician and make sure that you are getting all the vitamins and nutrients that you need to keep your body functioning well. Only a doctor is capable of truly evaluating your body's overall health and wellness, and I cannot emphasize enough how important it is to consult with them and keep them in the picture for your overall health.

There will also be days when it seems that cutting down on the calories and maintaining strength seems to be difficult. Well, it can even go beyond that – it could be depressing. When such days come, it would not hurt to have a cheat day. You can even make it a weekly cheat day if you want to. It would not only do your mind and emotions wonders, but it would also help you stabilize your thyroid, insulin, and leptin hormones so that they can recover more quickly on the next round. However, make sure that you do diet breaks in the latter part of your fat loss project, where you have less fat to lose. Otherwise, it can be difficult for you to go back to your fat loss routine.

You should also be able to control your appetite without depriving you of your joys of eating. Think of the food that you want as a reward. You can actually eat what you want on days that you are training, or scheduled to do a lot of work, as long as your activities are sufficient to burn the calories consumed. You can go back to taking in fewer calories during your rest days. This is called calorie cycling, which is essential to making sure that you have enough energy during your busy days. It is also needed to make you feel happy and satisfied during the entire fat loss regimen, without failing to get the results that you want.

Essentially, losing fat is easy to do as long as you can manage and maintain your daily activities. Choosing to trim body fat according to a caloric deficit works because it allows you to create a certain harmony between what your body needs and what you personally want. It is, in effect, a better way to practice the law of thermodynamics.

One Last Piece Of Advice To Get You Started!

Lastly I want to help you to get a rough idea of how many calories your body needs to maintain its current body weight. If you go to www.google.com or any other search engine and type in the phrase "maintenance calorie calculator" you will find a bunch of different sites that have this type of calculator. It will ask you a few questions and give you a rough idea of how many calories your body currently is burning, this way you will get a pretty good idea of your daily calorie maintenance level. Once you have this level figured out, you can use this as a guideline in your weight loss journey. Since your goal is losing fat you might start off by eating slightly less than this level for a while and track your progress. If you aren't reaching your goals in a period of a few months then you might want to decrease the calories further. One thing to keep in mind is that people tend to overdo the restrictions, just start of by restricting a small amount of calories and then track and re-adjust for progress. Many health professionals tend to recommend losing about 1 - 2 lbs per week, but this is different for everyone and you will need to consult with your doctor for specific advice. Remember the slower you lose the weight, the better chance of maintaining your hard earned muscle so don't try to do it too fast, and just remember this is a lifestyle not a diet.

Conclusion

Thank you again for purchasing this book!

I hope this book was able to help you understand the truth about fat loss and how to accomplish whatever fitness goals you might have.

The next step is to get started implementing these principles and strategies so you can become who you dream to be!

Also, if you know of anyone else that could benefit from the information presented in this book, then please tell them about it.

Finally, if you enjoyed this book, please take the time to share your thoughts and post a review on Amazon. It'd be greatly appreciated!

Thank you and good luck!

Preview Of:

<u>Intermittent Fasting Diet</u>

Lose Fat In 7 Days Intermittent Fasting!

.

Introduction

I want to thank you and congratulate you for purchasing the book, *"Intermittent Fasting Diet - Lose Fat in 7 Days Intermittent Fasting!"*.

This book contains proven steps and strategies on how Intermittent Fasting can not only help you lose fat rapidly, but keep it off for life!

Have you been working out consistently? Eating the recommended 4-6 meals each day? And still, you are unable to reveal your six pack and glutes to the world?

You are not alone. For years supplement companies, fitness magazines, bodybuilders, fitness trainers, health gurus, and many others have been all telling the same advice to lose fat and gain muscle. Their solution for your fitness goals - Eat 4-6 miniature chipmunk sized meals, do lots of weight training, and even more cardio. So, the time is now to ask yourself one simple question, "How's that working out for ya?".

If you don't feel too good about your fitness results, and really want to see that six pack, lean muscular physique, then you are reading the right book. The time is now to try the most revolutionary new diet, which I would rather refer to as a lifestyle - Intermittent Fasting!

Thanks again for purchasing this book, I hope you enjoy it!

Chapter 1 - Intermittent Fasting And Its Benefits

Intermittent fasting is markedly different from any other diet plan that you may have tried in the past. Most weight loss plans espoused by fitness gurus will tell you to control the amount you eat while keeping a close watch on the kinds of food that you do consume, usually in combination with a rigorous exercise routine. You know this: you've done the cardio, lifted the weights, run the miles, and eaten 6 small meals a day, all the while assiduously avoiding unhealthy fats and unnecessary carbohydrates.

But you are probably reading this book because this system just doesn't work for you – in fact, it has probably left you tired, crabby, and frustrated, with nothing to show for your hard work but a few insignificant inches shed from your waistline and some mad food cravings that are proving harder and harder to ignore.

This is not to say that typical diet programs don't work. After all, there's a reason why they have their staunch advocates. But the fact remains that for most people, it is much more effective – and much easier – to control when they eat, instead of what they eat and the portions thereof.

That's what intermittent fasting, also known as IF, is all about. To put it in the very simplest terms, when you adopt this lifestyle, you will only eat during a certain period of time daily, and go entirely without food, which is the fasting bit,for the rest of the day. That's all there is to it. And, once you consider the amount of time that there actually is between meals, you'll see that it isn't hard at all.

There is no denying that exercise and healthy eating are important (you can't hope to get that six-pack if you live on fast food burgers and stay on the couch all day, but more on that later), but intermittent fasting can work wonders on its own. Before we go on to the nitty-gritty of this fitness lifestyle, let's take a look at the unique benefits that it has to offer.

Better Weight Control and Faster Fat Loss

Since shedding pounds and losing inches are the most conspicuous signs of success of any diet program – not to mention your most likely objective when you start dieting –we'll start here. Intermittent fasting is exceptionally effective at helping you lose fat since it eases your body into a situation where it starts burning fat stores for energy. And since this will happen every single day that you go through a period of fasting, you will lose fat faster and have better control over your body weight than if you stick to counting calories.

Elimination of Pesky Food Cravings

One of the major trials for any dieter is the craving for snacks and sweets, and, admittedly, those will still be there when you start intermittent fasting. Once you get into the habit, however, you'll find that your pesky food cravings aren't troubling you as much, and soon you just won't feel them anymore. Scientists theorize that this is due to fasting bringing the level of your body's ghrelin, otherwise known as the "hunger hormone", down to normal, so you don't continually feel the urge to snack.

Reduced Oxidation with Boosted Autophagy

Oxidative stress caused by free radicals in your system can really take its toll on your body's cells. The damage done by free radicals to DNA, RNA, proteins, and lipids is known to advance the effects of aging and disease. Going on an intermittent fasting diet will help combat this by boosting autophagy, or the process by which cellular waste is recycled by your body. This helps your cells get rid of the trash, so to speak, so that they can continue to function optimally, allowing you to better withstand stress, disease, and aging.

A Healthier Nervous System and Mental Clarity

Though it is commonly believed that fasting will leave you weak and unable to think, nothing could be further from the truth. Intermittent fasting has actually been shown to enhance memory and learning, as well as helping to improve your disposition in life. This is because periodic fasting boosts the production of brain-derived neurotrophic factor (BDNF), a hormone that prevents the degradation of the neurons in your brain while stimulating the growth of new neurons. A boost in the neurotransmitter serotonin also happens, which leads to better moods and improved learning ability.

Enjoyable Longevity

While any sort of health and fitness regime has the long-term aim of prolonging your life, one of the main attractions of intermittent fasting for many people is that it promotes enjoyable longevity. Good health shouldn't mean giving up good food, or spending the rest of your long life obsessively counting calories. Intermittent fasting is a lifestyle that allows you to eat the way you like (up to a point!) while staying fit. In addition to that, scientific studies have shown that fasting can increase an animal's lifespan without retarding their growth, which is not the case for diets that focus on caloric restriction.

Thanks For Previewing My Exiting Book Entitled:

"Intermittent Fasting Diet – Lose Fat In 7 Days Intermittent Fasting!"

To purchase this book, simply go to the Amazon Kindle store and simply search:

"INTERMITTENT FASTING"

Then just scroll down until you see my book. You will know it is mine because you will see my name "Chris Smith" underneath the title.

Alternatively, you can visit my author page on Amazon to see this book and other work I have done. Thanks so much, and please don't forget your free bonuses

DON'T LEAVE YET! - CHECK OUT YOUR FREE BONUSES BELOW!

Free Bonus Offer: Get Free Access To The LiveFitVIP.com VIP Newsletter!

Once you enter your email address you will immediately get free access to this awesome newsletter!

But wait, right now if you join now for free you will also get free access to the "The 7 Keys To Body Transformation" free EBook!

To claim both your FREE VIP NEWSLETTER MEMBERSHIP and your FREE BONUS eBook on THE 7 KEYS TO BODY TRANSFORMATION!

Just Go To:

www.liveFitVIP.com

www.ingramcontent.com/pod-product-compliance
Lightning Source LLC
Chambersburg PA
CBHW070941290526
45795CB00003B/1100